C000142347

THE GASTRIC B᾽

A Practical Guide To Medications, Surgery, Recuperation, Complications, Risk And Expected Weight Loss; Including Dietary Guidelines

Thomas Cornett

TABLE OF CONTENT

CHAPTER ONE

Introduction

Weight reduction medical procedure was created utilizing two unique methodologies. One of these methodologies utilized procedures of limitation that constrained the admission of calories while the other concentrated on strategies of malabsorption that confined the measure of calories consumed by the body.

The first of these endeavors was the jejuno-ilial sidesteps by A.J. Kremen in 1954, which focused on the last of the two methodologies. In any case, this surgery brought about dietary inadequacies. The circumvent segment of digestive organs was excessively serious.

Because of these endeavors, a wide cluster of combinatorial techniques were created, including Duodenal Switch, Bilio Pancreatic Diversion, and Gastric Bypass.

These strategies didn't depend entirely on malabsorption; they likewise used prohibitive procedures, making a littler usable stomach. By consolidating both malabsorption and limitation, specialists had the option to sidestep a littler segment of the digestive organs. This decreased the danger of healthful insufficiencies from the detour while the diminished stomach size truly restricted the sum a patient could eat.

In 1967, the primary Gastric Bypass medical procedure was performed by Ito and Mason at the University of Iowa. This methodology was then adjusted throughout the years into its present structure.

This medical procedure is known as Roux-En-Y Gastric Bypass (RYGP). There are two different ways to play out this medical procedure: the open entry point strategy and the laproscopic technique, which utilizes 5 little cuts to lessen post-employable agony and speed recuperation.

There are two different ways to perform Roux-En-Y Gastric Bypass; open and laparoscopic. The laparoscopic method altogether diminishes post-usable agony and abbreviates the length of your emergency clinic remain.

The present laparoscopic gastric detour has been performed a huge number of times. Its results have been contemplated, its dangers and advantages assessed, and it's frequently secured by protection.

It's an amazing weight reduction arrangement and ought to be truly considered by anybody keen on bariatric medical procedure.

Gastric detour has truly been the most famous bariatric method (Bariatric Surgery Data Management and Reporting Worldwide). Since 2011 gastric sleeve medical procedure has developed rapidly in ubiquity and in 2015 is the most well known bariatric medical procedure alternative (to a great extent the aftereffect of Lap

Bands losing piece of the pie). Be that as it may, this ought not detract from the benefits of gastric detour medical procedure. It is still broadly acknowledged as the 'highest quality level' for bariatric medical procedure. Here's the reason:

• You will get more fit. By and large, you will lose 70% of your overabundance body weight in the initial year and a half after medical procedure.

• This study shows 77.5% of abundance weight reduction following year and a half. (Diary Of Obesity, 2013)

You won't have the option to eat huge suppers (limited pocket/stomach size).

You will become ill from eating an excessive amount of sugar and additionally carbs (dumping condition).

You will retain less calories from food (circumvent digestion tracts).

You will improve and additionally dispose of type 2 diabetes.

Prescription for hypertension as well as elevated cholesterol might be disposed of.

Your hormones may alter from critical weight reduction, expanding testosterone and improving digestion. (ASMBS)

Long haul weight reduction achievement – most investigations show that 90% of patients keep up at any rate half of overabundance weight reduction after medical procedure.

When you shed pounds and lessen drugs it gets simpler to work out. On the off chance that you can actualize customary exercise alongside a sound eating regimen, you may lose more than the normal overabundance weight reduction recorded previously.

Narrative, you will have more vitality, more certainty, and feel better after gastric detour medical procedure. These advantages are difficult to quantify however this examination shows 95% of patients announced an improved personal satisfaction 1 year after medical procedure.

The night prior to your medical procedure, you should quit eating. Attempt to unwind, scrub down, and spotlight on the reasons why you decided to have medical procedure. Dread and apprehensions are totally typical.

Upon the arrival of medical procedure, don't eat or drink anything (counting water or espresso) except if your specialist or anesthesiologist explicitly gives you authorization. At the point when you show up at the emergency clinic, you will be conceded and should round out desk work including assents. You'll meet the pre-operation nursing staff, your anesthesiologist and frequently your circling medical attendant (the medical caretaker that will be with you in the OR). On the off chance that you have concerns don't be hesitant to pose inquiries.

You will at that point change into your medical clinic outfit. You may likewise be solicited to wear a couple from graduated pressure stockings that are uniquely intended to forestall any blood coagulations from happening. Most offices will give against tension drug. An IV will at that point be embedded into your arm so anti-toxins might be regulated and intravenous liquids and drugs have an immediate way to your circulation system. The IV will stay until you are released.

You will at that point go into the working room, and clingy cushions will be set on your chest to screen your pulse. A breathing apparatus will be set all over and afterward sedation will be managed through the IV. You'll tally again from 10 and wake up in recuperation.

CHAPTER TWO

Recuperation

After Surgery

Recuperation time will rely upon the size of the cut made. On the off chance that you had laparoscopic gastric detour medical procedure performed, you will probably remain in the emergency clinic for 2 to 3 days. On the off chance that your medical procedure turned into open method (greater entry point) recuperation and your emergency clinic stay may last more.

The territory of the cuts will be sore in the days following medical procedure. In the emergency clinic this is handily dealt with prescription. Your specialist will probably have you stand and walk the equivalent day of your medical procedure. This helps expel any gas left over from the insufflations air used to grow your midsection and give space to work) utilized during your system. You will probably be approached to stroll around the clinic floor in any event multiple times day by day after medical procedure.

Numerous emergency clinics presently have understanding controlled absence of pain (PCA). This is a system that permits you to press fasten and direct agony prescription for yourself.

Your specialist will visit with you two or multiple times after medical procedure and before you are released. Ensure you have and comprehend the release directions just as any solutions as well as prescriptions that you will require once home.

Getting back

It's acceptable to be home. But on the other hand it's somewhat terrifying. You're on your own at this point.

Take Your Pain Medication

You will be sore and the touchiness/torment may deteriorate before it shows signs of improvement.

The specialist has recommended you torment prescription. Try not to hold back to get it from the drug store. Have a friend or family member get it for you or get it on your route home from the emergency clinic. Accept it as endorsed. Torment prescriptions can cause blockage. Your release directions ought to incorporate rules for dealing with clogging during your initial hardly any weeks after medical procedure.

Your primary care physician will anticipate that you should walk at whatever point conceivable however don't try too hard. You'll be extremely worn out. Keep in mind, you haven't eaten anything in a couple of days and simply had significant medical procedure. So once more, don't try too hard in those first weeks yet stroll around the house much of the time.

Hydrate

Drink your water. Drying out turns into a genuine hazard after medical procedure Food gives us a considerable lot of our day by day water. Without food, you should give close consideration to your water admission to forestall lack of hydration. Top off a huge water bottle with all the water you'll requirement for the afternoon and begin tasting. Try not to utilize a straw to drink your water. It's anything but difficult to drink an excess of excessively fast and you hazard gulping air which squeezes your new stomach. Little tastes, no straws, throughout the day.

Rest

You may have plans of promptly beginning activity, cleaning the house, sorting out and assisting the family. You should rest. You'll be worn out. You'll have the opportunity to clean and sort out and everything else except for those initial hardly any weeks, plan on resting.

On the off chance that you have a chair you may feel more great resting in it. A slight slope can mitigate a portion of the agony in your mid-region and lessen the danger of acid reflux. On the off chance that you don't have a chair, have a couple of additional cushions at home.

Action

Hacking is frequently urged to extend your lungs and raise any liquids that may stay after medical procedure. Be that as it may, hacking harms after medical procedure. Numerous specialists suggest utilizing a hack pad. Hold this tight to your stomach when you want to hack. It will forestall enormous developments in your mid-region and diminish torment.

Continuously adhere to your release guidelines. It is commonly prescribed to not lift anything weighing more than 15 pounds for in any event six or seven weeks. Continue strolling. Increment your separation as your body permits it. Test out the steps once you feel like it however go slowly. In the event that a specific movement is excessively troublesome or causes torment, don't drive it.

Entry points

Try not to absorb a shower. It is regularly prescribed to hold up until your first follow-up arrangement before showering. It's significant that your cuts have the opportunity to recuperate and remain clean. A little redness around the entry points is ordinary. Waste, discharge, and putrid smells at the entry point destinations ought to be accounted for to your specialist.

Follow-up Appointments

Your first follow-up arrangement is about seven days after your medical procedure; on the off chance that you have skin staples they might be expelled right now. About a month later, you will return for your second development, and about month from that point forward, you will return for your third. Most specialists will at that point need to see you four months after the fact (which is an a large portion of a year after your medical procedure) and afterward 6th months from that point forward, which would be a year after your medical procedure was finished. Recollect that these are just surmised occasions for your subsequent arrangements. Various specialists may have various calendars, or your condition may require more visits.

Try not to skirt your subsequent arrangements. Try not to be reluctant to share your battles and worries after medical procedure. Your specialist can't assist you with refocusing in the event that you are not legitimate with the person in question.

After your yearly exam, most specialists will need to see you once per year. You will get medicine tops off and have routine blood work performed at every one of these yearly visits. The blood work guarantees you are not supplement lacking.

CHAPTER THREE

Diet

Your bariatric program ought to have hearty, straightforward eating regimen rules and you ought to be exceptionally acquainted with them before medical procedure. Preparing your home with suggested food items and protein shakes is prompted.

Pre-Op Liquid Diet

Up to 14 days earlier medical procedure your specialist or dietitian will ask that you start a pre-operation diet. The pre-operation diet for gastric detour commonly resembles this:

•   5 to 7 fluid feast substitution shakes every day. High protein, low carb shakes are suggested. The Baritastic Store has various famous dinner substitution shakes.

• 64 to 96 ounces of water for every day. Utilize the Bariatric Surgery App to follow this.

• Some specialists may permit a little bit of vegetables day by day.

The objective of the pre-operation diet is to recoil the size of your liver so it's simpler for your specialist to get to your stomach during medical procedure. The pre-operation diet is intense yet significant. You will be eager, bleary eyed, and irritable for the primary couple of days. By day three you should begin to feel better as your body begins to consume fat rather than carbs as your essential vitality source.

Post-Op Dietary Guidelines

An exacting eating routine should now be followed for a few reasons. Your stomach is currently a lot littler and recouping. Your digestion tracts have been cut and re-steered. There are staples in both of these regions holding the tissue together. It's essential to not put any unjustifiable weight on this tissue while it's mending. Huge dinners, sinewy food, carbonated drinks can prompt a staple line spill. Try not to hazard a genuine complexity. Follow your post-operation diet!

There are four periods of the post-operation diet:

1. Clear Liquids

2. Pureed Foods and Protein Shakes

3. Soft Foods

4. Solid Foods

Stage One: Liquids

For about seven days after medical procedure, just certain fluids are to be tasted gradually at the pace of two ounces for every hour. Most dietitians and specialists will suggest things like water and without sugar jello just as sans fat stock and sans fat milk the graph underneath shows an ordinary fluid eating routine for the primary week after medical procedure.

Stage Two: Pureed Foods and Protein Shakes

Your primary care physician or dietitian will decide when the subsequent stage will start. For the following week or two, you will have the option to expend pureed nourishments a few times for the duration of the day in little segments. During this stage, center around eating gradually every little segment of delicate food ought to be expended over a brief period. Eating every dinner gradually, taking in any event 30 minutes for every supper, ought to stay an objective through the entirety of the post-employable stages and past. The Baritastic application has a food clock that is helpful for this reason.

Most dietitians and specialists will prescribe a day by day admission of 60 to 70 grams of protein for each day and around 64 ounces of the sorts of fluids expended in stage one. Fat, sugar, caffeine, and carbonated refreshments ought to be kept away from. Your dietitian or specialist will likely permit you to expend egg whites, protein shakes, non-fat curds, and creamed soups with any pieces skimmed out. Hold up in any event 30 minutes when eating before drinking.

Stage Three: Soft Foods

During this piece of your post-operation diet plan, you will step by step start to include food substances with more surfaces. This stage will generally last from one to three weeks, contingent upon the suggestions of your primary care physician or dietitian.

In this stage, you will have the option to expend some lean meats and vegetables that are sufficiently delicate to be handily squashed with a fork, and your healthful objectives will continue as before as they were in stage two. A limited quantity of fat may be permitted.

Suggested delicate nourishments will likely incorporate things, for example, fish, egg whites, tofu, without fat curds, sans fat cheddar, canned fish, and canned or destroyed chicken mollified with water. The vegetables that may be May recommended incorporate avocados, pounded green beans, steamed carrots, and squash. Bananas will likely be permitted too. Notwithstanding, bananas have a high sugar content. Break your banana into scaled down bits and just eat a nibble or two out of one sitting.

Stage Four: Solids

This is the last phase of your post-operation diet plain. Go moderate. Presenting new nourishments excessively fast can cause difficult gas, swelling, indigestion and dumping condition. Present each new food in turn. Hold up a day prior presenting another new food.

The objective in stage four is to re-present solid nourishments in little parts. It is still prescribed to begin with milder nourishments and continuously work into chewy and stringy nourishments.

Make sure to take as much time as necessary eating and keep on biting each chomp of food well.

Monitor your protein and guarantee you are eating well vegetables as your essential starch source. Avoid' garbage' starches, for example, refined sugar, pasta, rice, bread, chips, and so on.

You should now have the option to diminish your suppers every day to three little, supplement thick dinners (protein and vegetable). Supplement with your protein shakes and remember required nutrients and enhancements.

Your all out caloric admission will in the end arrive at 1,000 to 1,500 calories for every day except don't constrain it. Certain nourishments are hard for your body to process. Include them gradually and in little segments. These nourishments incorporate corn, nuts, beans, meat, pork, shellfish, and grapes.

CHAPTER FOUR

Dumping Syndrome

Your body has a wellbeing valve known as the pylorus. It keeps food from entering the small digestion tracts until it has been separated by gastric juices. The pylorus is skirted during gastric detour medical procedure. After gastric detour medical procedure your stomach may rashly dump its substance into the small digestion tracts. This is called 'dumping condition.'

Dumping condition causes stomach inconvenience, squeezing, and expanded pulse, looseness of the bowels, dazedness, and queasiness. It is entirely awkward. Refined sugars are the essential driver of dumping condition yet eating excessively or too quick can likewise cause dumping disorder.

Dumping disorder isn't acceptable. What's more, when you've encountered it, you will attempt to dodge it no matter what.

Be that as it may, dumping condition fortifies your dietary rules. On the off chance that you don't eat little suppers gradually, decrease or wipe out basic starches and refined sugars, you may encounter dumping condition. This is a solid helper to avoid undesirable nourishments.

Early dumping is a sort of dumping condition that happens not exactly thirty minutes after a feast, and its manifestations incorporate perspiring, sickness, cramps, looseness of the bowels, wooziness, swelling, and spewing. Late dumping is another type of dumping condition that happens following an hour or more after a dinner and incorporates most the manifestations of early dumping just as appetite and swooning.

Nutrients and Supplements

After gastric detour medical procedure your new stomach will limit the measure of food you can eat. Your avoided digestive organs will likewise lessen the measure of nutrients and minerals assimilated.

It is important to take nutrients and enhancements for an amazing remainder after medical procedure.

It is significant that you take the necessary nutrients and enhancements after medical procedure for an amazing remainder.

Multivitamin

You should take a couple of multivitamins (contingent upon the kind of nutrient) during the second or third period of your dietary arrangement (consistently check with your specialist). These multivitamins ought to be taken with suppers, and this training should proceed for an amazing remainder.

After medical procedure it tends to be hard to swallow pills. You might need to consider nutrient patches. As usual, check with your bariatric specialist to guarantee these nutrients address your issues.

Calcium Citrate

Calcium citrate (for the most part something like 500 mg multiple times/day) is a significant dietary enhancement. It ought to be taken with suppers yet not simultaneously as the multivitamin in light of the fact that the iron in the multivitamin will meddle with the ingestion of the calcium. A few specialists and dietitians may need you to begin calcium citrate in stage two and others may suggest you start it in stage three.

Note: Calcium citrate ingests far superior to calcium carbonate after gastric detour medical procedure. Calcium carbonate isn't suggested.

Nutrient D3

In either stage two or stage three, you will be required to start supplementation with Vitamin D3. You will presumably be told to take roughly 500 IU twice day by day. These measurements ought to be taken with your calcium supplementation.

Nutrient B12

After your medical procedure, your stomach related framework will not, at this point have the option to process satisfactory measures of nutrient B12. 500 to 1,200 mcg of nutrient B12 in sublingual structure is suggested. By taking it sublingually (under your tongue) it is straightforwardly retained into the circulation system and doesn't need to enter the stomach related lot where its bioavailability is diminished.

You additionally have the alternative of getting month to month infusions of B12. You can play out these infusions yourself or have them controlled by your primary care physician at your month to month tests.

Iron

Iron is invested in the duodenum, which is the piece of the small digestive system that is avoided after gastric detour medical procedure. Accordingly, your body is not, at this point ready to ingest satisfactory measures of iron. The iron got in multivitamins may not be sufficient, and your PCP may need you to start iron supplementation. This is especially valid for females during their month to month cycle.

Your primary care physician may likewise suggest that you additionally start taking nutrient C since it enables your body to all the more likely assimilate iron. The sum and sort of iron to be taken will likewise be controlled by your PCP. Numerous patients are recommended 500 to 1,000 mg of natural iron every day. Ferrous fumarate and ferrous gluconate are the two most bioavailable types of iron supplementation.

Note that you would prefer not to take iron simultaneously as calcium since they meddle with one another's ingestion.

Would it be able to be stretched?

Indeed. The stomach is comprised of folds of tissue called rugae that extend an agreement to oblige food and fluid. The extending of the stomach might be incompletely liable for the sentiment of 'completion' after dinners.

On the off chance that you eat a huge dinner your stomach will stretch and, afterward contract. On the off chance that you keep on huge eat dinners; you may begin to feel like you 'require' a huge feast to get 'full.' This can make a pattern of eating totality, at that point eating before your stomach has completely contracted and feeling like you need increasingly more food to feel 'full.'

The following are a couple of tips to help forestall extending your stomach after gastric detour.

• Do not eat until you feel 'full.' Eat a foreordained estimated dinner that is proper for how out of sight are from medical procedure.

- If the measure of food on your plate is more than the size of your clench hand, you are likely eating excessively.

Try not to drink and eat simultaneously. Both fluid and food end up in your stomach. Separate fluids and food by at any rate 30 minutes.

- Don't drink carbonated refreshments. The air pockets can squeeze your stomach.

Eat gradually and bite well.

CHAPTER FIVE

Expected Weight Loss

You can hope to lose between 60 to 80 percent of your overabundance weight from gastric detour medical procedure. The greater part of the weight reduction happens in the initial year and a half after medical procedure. There is a hazard for weight recapture after medical procedure, yet gastric detour medical procedure has outstanding amongst other long haul weight reduction profiles when contrasted with other essential medicines for horrible heftiness.

Gastric detour is a device to get your weight down to a solid level. When your weight is down it's dependent upon you to actualize solid propensities that keep up or improve the weight reduction. The following are a couple of sound propensities that will help continue or potentially improve your general weight reduction after medical procedure.

- Eat three little supplement thick dinners every day.

- Exercise 3 to 5 times each week.

- Journal what you eat. The Baritastic application is incredible for this.

- Follow-up with your specialist as suggested. You'd be astonished at what numbers of individuals don't return following a half year.

- Attend bolster gatherings.

- Make companions, join discussions.

- Get your relatives to execute a sound way of life.

In the event that you'd prefer to ascertain your normal weight reduction after gastric detour, you can utilize the number cruncher underneath. Note that this number cruncher depends on the normal overabundance weight reduction of 70% after gastric detour medical procedure. You can lose more on the off chance that you the computations depend on normal weight reduction per system. To lose the normal measure of weight, you'll have to follow your specialist's pre-employable and post-usable rules.

Long haul diet and exercise changes alongside other propensity changes can prompt weight reduction that surpasses the midpoints utilized in these estimations.

On normal gastric detour patients lose about 70% (Bariatric Surgery, A Systemic Review and Meta Analysis, 2004) of their overabundance weight. Gastric sleeve patients lose about 60% of their abundance weight. Also, Lap Band patients lose about half of their overabundance weight.

Droopy Skin

Droopy or free skin is regular subsequent to losing loads of weight rapidly. Notwithstanding the methodology or diet used to shed pounds, on the off chance that you are extremely chubby and shed pounds rapidly, you may have droopy skin. This is a reality.

There are systems to evacuate skin after gastric detour medical procedure. At times, these are secured by protection.

Over numerous years, your skin extended as your body developed. While skin has some flexibility, it will probably not completely fix to coordinate your new littler body.

Age assumes a job. More youthful patients will in general have greater flexibility in their skin. As we age our skin normally loses versatility. Furthermore, more youthful patients have regularly been overweight for a shorter measure of time. The skin can 'skip' back snappier in these patients.

The aggregate sum of weight lost assumes a job. On the off chance that you lose 200 to 300 pounds, you will probably have additional skin. On the off chance that you lose 50 to 100 lbs, you will probably have less. What's more, in case you're youthful, you may have next to no if any free skin.

This appears to be quite evident however it's significant. Setting legitimate desires will help with your general fulfillment and bliss after medical procedure. The objective of bariatric medical procedure is to improve your wellbeing by lessening the comorbidities related with corpulence. This is certifiably not a restorative method.

The following are a couple of things you can do that may help diminish (not dispense with) droopy skin after gastric detour medical procedure. These are recounted.

• Hydrate. Drink a lot of liquids to keep your skin sound.

• Moisturize.

• Exercise utilizing loads.

•   Stretch. Yoga or workout can assist work with yearning fit muscles which can make a more 'conditioned' look.

•   Eat leafy foods.

•   Use sunscreen day by day. Sun can harm the skin and may decrease versatility.

Enthusiastic and Mindset Changes

Get ready for passionate changes after gastric detour medical procedure. Uneven characters of estrogen, progesterone and testosterone are identified with misery (Holtorfmed). Getting more fit changes your parity of testosterone estrogen and thyroid creation (Surgery for Obesity and Related Diseases, 2007).

This can be a much needed development as expanded thyroid hormone can build vitality in patients with subclinical hypothyroidism. In any case, getting in shape rapidly after medical procedure may adjust testosterone and estrogen levels. These hormonal changes can cause a scope of troublesome feelings. Despondency, outrage, sentiments of misery, and lament are normal during the primary year after medical procedure.

Expecting and getting ready for these enthusiastic changes can help lessen their effect. Go to help gatherings and set up your loved ones. After some time, your hormones and feelings will discover solidness.

It's additionally critical to take note of that numerous patients have medical procedure and never experience enthusiastic unsteadiness.

CHAPTER SIX

Gastric Bypass Risks

While the advantages of gastric detour are amazing, the dangers should be weighed cautiously.

Significant Complications

Significant difficulties can bring about death. The danger of death after gastric detour is under 1% as indicated by most examinations. The death rate (demise) from gastric detour medical procedure is like the mortality related with basic surgeries, for example, gallbladder expulsion.

Pneumonic Embolism

This condition is caused when blood coagulation structures after medical procedure and afterward goes to your lungs where it forestalls appropriate blood/gas trade. Its indications incorporate chest torment, windedness, stun, swooning, quick pulse, and passing. Most occasions of this condition can be treated with blood thinners (anticoagulants); in any case, if the condition is dangerous, thrombolytics (uncommon drugs that are fit for separating enormous clusters) or medical procedure might be required. Staple Line Leaks

Holes for the most part happen when the tissue holding the staples breaks down or when the staples themselves fizzle. This makes a gap where the substance of your inside as well as stomach spill into your midsection. These breaks can frequently be fixed on the off chance that they are found early enough. Indications incorporate serious agony, expanded pulse, and fever.

There are two essential ways that specialists will check for releases; a pocket test utilizing air while searching for bubbles or infusing color and afterward searching for the color in the mid-region. Minor holes are commonly treated by resting the stomach and taking care of the patient with an IV; in any case, once in a while medical procedure is required for more serious holes.

Little Bowel Obstruction

Little entrail impediments may happen not long after medical procedure or years after the fact. Side effects incorporate stomach torment and growing just as retching. An analysis can be made with either a CAT output or medical procedure. Treatment of this condition may require medical procedure.

Different Risks and Downsides

Pregnancy

Ladies of childbearing age should hold up year and a half after medical procedure before getting pregnant.

Sickness

Sickness is a typical event for some individuals who have had gastric detour medical procedure. What's more, your odds of encountering this condition are around 70 percent. As a rule, sickness is brought about by resistance with the dietary rules given to you by your PCP Making sure to eat the right things, not drinking while at the same time eating, and biting your food appropriately will decrease sickness.

Lack of hydration

This condition happens when your liquids have been exhausted. The most ideal approach to forestall lack of hydration is to taste a lot of liquids for the duration of the day. This is especially significant the main week after medical procedure when you can just take little tastes. Top off a container with 64 ounces of water and gradually taste like clockwork.

Acid reflux

Acid reflux is normally joined by distress in the upper bit of your mid-region. This condition is treated by drinking just liquids for a specific timeframe and totally maintaining a strategic distance from oily nourishments. In the event that adjustments in your eating regimen neglect to mitigate this condition, acid neutralizers might be utilized as type of treatment. However, as usual, counsel your primary care physician before self-sedating.

Wound Site Infection

Wound site diseases have a wide scope of frequency (from 1.5% to 20%) and it might be identified with the strategy used to make the gastro-jejunostomy (stomach to digestive system anastamosis). Whenever treated early, twisted site diseases can be made do with anti-infection agents. Open strategies have a higher danger of wound site contaminations.

Ulcers

After gastric detour medical procedure there is a danger of ulcers. Smokers and individuals who utilize certain meds are at a higher danger of creating post-employable ulcers. The following is a rundown of regular drugs to stay away from after medical procedure. This rundown isn't extensive. Your release guidelines ought to incorporate a total rundown of drugs to keep away from. What's more, don't smoke. Smoking expands your danger of ulcers.

- Alka-seltzer

- Ibuprofen

- Excedrin

- Motrin

- Pepto-bismol

Different Complications

There are different confusions that are not talked about in this article. They extend in seriousness and incorporate injuries, tissue ischemia, inside hernias, and gastric reflux (indigestion) among others.

What Does It All Mean?

Gastric detour is viewed as a sheltered methodology. The normal confusion rate is 5.9% in the initial 30 days after laparoscopic gastric detour medical procedure (MBSQAIP). What's more, the danger of death is like the danger of death with basic surgeries, for example, gallbladder expulsion.

CHAPTER SEVEN

Conclusion

Gastric detour medical procedure is an all around read compelling treatment for sullen weight. While there are new surgeries for weight reduction, none have the drawn out information, great outcomes and wellbeing profile that gastric detour has more than once appeared. Gastric detour remains the 'Highest quality level' for weight reduction medical procedure and ought to be firmly considered by all bariatric medical procedure up-and-comers.

Printed in Great Britain
by Amazon

58459568R00031